Kegel Exercise

for

Women

*Complete guide for postpartum recovery &
enhanced sexual function*

Kegel Exercise for Women

Written by

Gilbert predmore

Index

Chapter 1

Introduction to the Pelvic Floor and Postpartum Recovery

You will feel a lot of love and joy for your new baby during the postpartum period, but your feelings may also go up and down, leaving you confused, nervous, or even sad. This time can make you feel a lot of different feelings, such as happiness and love, tiredness and weariness, worry and anxiety, sadness and disappointment, loneliness and isolation, frustration and anger, and the need to get professional help if you need it.

Join a support group, talk to someone you trust, don't be afraid to ask for help, take care of yourself, and get professional help if you need it to get through the emotional waves. Not only should you admire your body, which carried and birthed a new life, but you should also accept and understand it as it heals and gets used to its new shape.

The journey of becoming a mother starts with big changes in the body. Not only should you admire your body, but you should also accept and understand it as it heals and gets used to its new shape. Going through these changes can make you feel a lot of different things.

From having a belly bump to not having one: your once-proud baby bump has flown away, leaving behind a soft, stretched canvas. Strengthen your pelvic floor muscles with Kegel movements to show appreciation for how strong and resilient your body is.

Separation of abdominal muscles is a normal event, not a flaw. Embrace gentle mending practices and workout changes to help your core muscles reunite.

Embrace healing, not competition: Comparison with pre-pregnancy pictures or famous standards are damaging and unrealistic. Recovery is personal, not a game. Focus on small wins, like regaining energy or getting into a comfortably supported pair of jeans. Celebrate your body's trip, not its goal.

Tips for good guidance include self-care routines, body praise practices, realistic standards, and self-love. Nourish your body with healthy foods, value sleep, and engage in activities that bring you joy. Look in the mirror with love, focus on your strengths, and recognize the beauty of your change. Set realistic goals and enjoy each milestone. Don't be afraid to ask for help and support from your healthcare provider or other moms.

Remember, the physical changes after childbirth are not flaws, but memories of your power and endurance. By accepting your body with kindness and understanding, you can handle this time with greater confidence and self-love. You are not alone on this journey, and your changed body is a witness to the amazing miracle you brought into the world.

The pelvic floor is an important part of the postpartum journey, giving support and control for the bladder, uterus, and rectum. These muscles, often ignored, play a significant role in avoiding problems like urine leakage, pelvic organ collapse, and pain during sex. Kegel movements can help regain strength and improve performance by squeezing and stretching these muscles.

Starting with Kegel movements includes finding your pelvic floor muscles, stopping pee midway, and starting with short squeezes, holding for a few seconds, and then easing. Gradually increase the length and strength of your squeezes as you get stronger.

Strong pelvic floor muscles not only improve core strength and stability, enhance sexual pleasure and feeling, ease lower back pain, and support healthy bowel movements. Consistency is key, so make Kegel movements a part of your daily practice.

A complete approach to pelvic floor health is important, including keeping a healthy weight, learning good posture, staying hydrated, reducing stress, and listening to your body. If you experience any pain or soreness during Kegel movements, ask your healthcare expert for personalized advice.

Embracing self-care is important for a good postpartum healing. Prioritize sleep, feed your body with healthy meals rich in fruits, veggies, and whole grains, move your body through gentle exercise, and practice breathing techniques to handle stress and anxiety. Set realistic goals for yourself, as healing takes time and you should be patient with yourself.
Embrace the changes in your body, focusing on accepting and enjoying your new form and strength rather than fixating on pre-pregnancy ideals. Ask for help from your partner, family, friends, and healthcare experts, as every woman heals at her own pace. Communicate and fight for yourself through open conversation, making regular checkups with your doctor or nurse, and getting professional help if required.

Educate yourself by reading books, articles, and online tools about postpartum healing, pelvic floor health, and baby care. Join a support group to provide mental support, shared experiences, and useful tips. Be your own champion by listening to your body and following your feelings.

The postpartum time is a chance for growth and change. By accepting self-care, setting realistic goals, speaking effectively, and seeking knowledge and support, you can strengthen your recovery and emerge stronger, healthier, and more confident than ever before. Remember, you are a fighter, a mother, and an example, and enjoy every win, big or small.

The pelvic floor muscles, often ignored but important for general well-being, play a major part in bladder control, core strength, sexual feeling, and overall pelvic health. They provide support and lift for the full core, taking pressure off shallow abdominal muscles and reducing lower back pain. When strong and toned, they work closely with deep core muscles to tighten and form an internal "brace," stopping leaking and supporting the body during quick moves.
A strong pelvic floor helps pull the spine into proper position, leading to better posture and reducing slouching or hunching, which can add to neck and shoulder pain. It also improves physical ability, helping people to work at their best. Kegel exercises and other pelvic floor awareness movements can help everyone, regardless of age or fitness level.

Recovering from childbirth involves not only physical healing but also recovering strength and control in key areas like the pelvic floor muscles. Kegel movements can be a great tool to help them bounce back. To build on this idea, describe Kegel movements as a positive and proactive way to regain control and strength after childbirth, stressing the benefits they offer, such as better bladder control, decreased chance of prolapse, and increased core stability.

Be inclusive, keep a calm and polite tone, praise body awareness, and support safety by contacting a healthcare professional before starting any exercise program, especially after childbirth. A strong pelvic floor can also be a powerful tool for improving sexual pleasure, but it's important to approach this subject with care and subtlety, considering the varied experiences and tastes of people.

Consider Kegel movements that target different muscle groups, adjust them using biofeedback or phone apps, gradually increase length and strength over time, and focus on mind-body links through yoga and Pilates. Meditation and breathwork can increase pelvic floor awareness and control, while imagination can improve involvement.

Healthy habits such as water, fiber-rich food, and stress management methods can help control stress and improve general pelvic health. By focusing on these key points, you can better understand and utilize the pelvic floor muscles for your general well-being and sexual pleasure.

The pelvic floor is an important part of the body, giving support, power, and pleasure. It is made of three paired muscles: ***the pubococcygeus, puborectalis, and iliococcygeus***. These muscles form a protective base for the pelvic organs, stopping them from prolapsing downward. They are multitaskers, playing a crucial part in bladder control, pelvic support, sexual function, childbirth, general well-being, and sports performance.

To take care of your pelvic floor, it is important to practice Kegel movements, keep a healthy weight, stay hydrated, handle stress, and listen to your body. Kegel movements involve squeezing and loosening the muscles, with 10-15 repeats, three times a day, gradually increasing length and strength. Maintaining a healthy weight can put pressure on the pelvic floor, while staying hydrated keeps the muscles working properly. Stress can tighten the pelvic floor, leading to pain, so relaxing methods like yoga or meditation can be helpful.

Understanding the structure and function of your pelvic floor muscles is the first step to unlocking their full potential. By practicing Kegel movements, choosing healthy habits, and listening to your body, you can strengthen your pelvic floor, improving your well-being and feeling all it has to offer.

There are three common postpartum pelvic floor issues: **weakness, incontinence, and diastasis recti**.

Diversity and equality should be recognized, as every woman's healing process is unique. Listen to your body, seek professional help if needed, and value your well-being. Remember, you are strong and robust, and by knowing your pelvic floor and taking positive steps, you can beat these challenges and recover your sense of power and confidence.

Kegel exercises are a crucial tool for postpartum healing, as they directly target the pelvic floor muscles, tightening them and boosting their strength and tone. These movements can improve bladder control, increase sexual function, lower the risk of prolapse, promote healing, regain body confidence, and be easily done anywhere, anytime.

Kegel movements are simple yet strong contractions that strengthen the muscles supporting the bladder, rectum, and uterus. They form the base of the hip and play a key role in different body processes. Strong pelvic floor muscles work in combination with core muscles to provide stability and support for the lower back and spine, helping prevent back pain, improve balance, and better exercise performance.

Better bowel control is another benefit of Kegel exercises, as strong pelvic floor muscles allow for better control over bowel movements, avoiding constipation and fecal leakage. Enhanced sexual performance can also be improved by improving blood flow and sensitivity.

Reduced urine leakage is another benefit of Kegel movements, as weak pelvic floor muscles add to various pelvic pain conditions, such as vulvodynia and endometriosis. Kegel movements can strengthen these muscles, giving relief from pain and soreness.

Postpartum recovery can be a difficult time for people, but Kegel movements can help regain their strength and tone, promoting faster healing and lowering pain associated with episiotomies or tears. It is important to discuss your doctor before starting Kegel movements, especially if you have any underlying health problems.

To reap the effects of Kegel movements, focus on strengthening and releasing the pelvic floor muscles, not the stomach or hip muscles. Be patient and steady, as it may take several weeks or even months to see noticeable effects.

By adding Kegel movements into your daily routine, you can reap numerous benefits for your physical and sexual health. These simple workouts can strengthen your core, improve bladder control, and even ease pain, making you feel your best from the inside out.

Some popular misunderstandings and worries about Kegel movements include:

1. Kegels are only for women.
2. Kegels are just "squeezing your butt."
3. Kegels won't work if you have had children.
4. Kegels won't stop urine leaks totally.
5. You might over-do it with Kegels.

To handle these misunderstandings and worries, try these tips:

1. Imagine pulling your pelvic floor muscles up and inward, like a lift.
2. Place a finger inside your vagina or near your rectum to feel the muscle spasms.

3. Listen to your body. Stop if you feel any pain or soreness. Aim for 3 sets of 10-15 contractions, 3 times a day, and gradually increase as allowed.

Consistency is key. Make Kegels part of your daily practice for best benefits.

Don't compare your progress to others. Everyone's pelvic floor is different, and improvement takes time. Consult your doctor for specific advice and rule out any underlying conditions. By handling these misunderstandings and concerns, you can approach Kegel movements with confidence and experience their numerous benefits for better pelvic health and general well-being.

Chapter 2

Mastering kegel Exercise for postpartum recovery

Your pelvic floor muscles are a group of muscles that form the base of your pelvis, like a net holding your bladder, rectum, and uterus. Strengthening these muscles can bring a variety of benefits, from better bladder control and sexual function to reduced pain and enhanced core stability. But the first step to receiving these gains is learning to spot and exercise these often-neglected muscles.

Finding Your Pelvic Floor:

There are several ways to identify your pelvic floor muscles, and finding the method that works best for you is key to good Kegel movements. Here are a few options:

The "Stop the Flow" Trick: Imagine you're in the middle of peeing and need to quickly stop the flow. The muscles you engage to do this are your pelvic floor muscles.

The Mirror, Mirror on the Wall: Lie down easily on your back with knees bent and feet flat on the floor. Relax your entire body and then picture pulling your pelvic floor muscles upward, as if trying to draw them towards your belly button. You might see a slight tightening or inward movement of your lower belly.

The Fingertip Test: For women, put a finger gently into your vagina. As you tighten your pelvic floor muscles, you should feel a small squeeze or lift around your finger. Again, focus on the internal muscles, not closing your vaginal hole.

Engaging Your Pelvic Floor:

Once you've found your pelvic floor muscles, it's time to learn how to tighten and rest them. Here's the basic Kegel exercise technique:

1. Squeeze: Imagine you're lifting your pelvic floor muscles up and inward, like an elevator. Hold the contraction for 3-5 seconds.
2. Relax: Completely release your pelvic floor muscles and let them return to their resting state. Hold the rest for 10 seconds.
3. Repeat: Aim for 10-15 repetitions of this squeeze-relax pattern, completing 3 sets throughout the day.

Strengthening your pelvic floor muscles with Kegel exercises can bring a multitude of benefits, but the journey isn't always smooth sailing. Let's address some common challenges and mistakes to help you handle your Kegel practice with confidence and effectiveness:

Challenge 1: Identifying and Isolating the Muscles

Mistake: Mistaking buttock or stomach movements for pelvic floor contact.

Tip: Focus on the internal feeling of lifting upward from the base of your hips, not squeezing your buttocks or tightening your belly. Imagine stopping the flow of pee midway to recognize the right muscles.

Challenge 2: Maintaining Consistent Practice

Mistake: Getting frustrated by slow progress or forgetting to do the exercises regularly.

Tip: Set notes on your phone, add Kegels into your daily routine while watching TV or reading, and track your progress with a chart or app to stay inspired. Celebrate small wins and remember, persistence is key!

Challenge 3: Performing Kegels Incorrectly

Mistake: Holding your breath, pulling, or pushing down instead of lifting up.

Tip: Breathe freely throughout the exercises, avoid stopping your breath, and focus on a smooth, controlled squeeze and release of your pelvic floor muscles. Imagine lifting an elevator, not pushing down on a handle.

Challenge 4: Experiencing Pain or Discomfort

Mistake: Pushing too hard, doing too many repeats, or ignoring pain signs.

Tip: Listen to your body! Stop if you feel any pain or soreness, and visit your doctor before restarting Kegels. Start with short, gentle movements and gradually increase strength as you get stronger.

Everyone's pelvic floor is different, and improvement takes time. Be patient and kind to yourself.With determination and the right method, you can beat challenges, avoid common mistakes, and enjoy the numerous benefits that Kegel movements have to offer for your general well-being

Although Kegel exercises have many advantages, not everyone responds well to a one-size-fits-all method. It's important to modify the workouts based on your unique demands and stage of recuperation in order to optimize their efficiency and guarantee safety. How to do it is as follows:

Problems with Bladder Control: To enhance bladder control and lessen leaks, concentrate on brief, rapid contractions (3-5 seconds) and full relaxation periods (10 seconds).

Enhancement: To improve sensitivity and blood flow during intercourse, use longer holds (8–10 seconds) with slower releases.

Postpartum Recovery: After speaking with your doctor, begin with mild contractions. As your body heals, progressively increase the force and length of the contractions.

Pelvic discomfort: Focus on calm, controlled motions and steer clear of harsh contractions when designing workouts that specifically target the muscles generating discomfort.

Choosing Exercises Based on Your Stage of Recovery:

Early Postpartum (First 6 Weeks): Perform gentle squeeze-and-hold exercises three times a day for five to ten seconds each, paying attention to correct technique and avoiding strain.

Mid-Postpartum (6–12 Weeks): Incorporate pulsing methods and gradually increase the length and intensity of contractions, aiming for 8–10 second holds.

Explore advanced Kegel exercises, such as "elevator" movements and variants that target certain muscle groups, in the **late postpartum** period (12+ weeks).

Your Kegel exercises should change as your workout regimen does to increase strength and endurance as well as to keep your pelvic floor muscles challenged and effective. Here's how to modify your regimen for the best outcomes:

Strategies for Progression:

- Lengthen Duration: As your muscles become stronger, progressively extend the time between each contraction (up to 10 seconds).
- Add Pulses: To improve muscular control and coordination, add brief, rapid pulses (squeeze-release-squeeze) after a complete contraction.
- Change situations: Kegel exercises should be performed in a variety of situations, including sitting, standing, laying down, and walking, to challenge your muscles.
- Include Challenges: To strengthen your pelvic floor muscles even more, use Kegel weights or vaginally implanted cones to increase resistance.

In general;

1. Start with Basic Kegels: do three sets of ten to fifteen repetitions, paused for three to five seconds each, three times a day.
2. Increase Duration Gradually: - Practice holding contractions for ten seconds.

3. Include Pulses and Variations: - Use short pulses and experiment with various placements.
4. Take Resistance Into Account: - If suitable, use Kegel weights or cones under the supervision of an expert.

Exercise modifications are essential for safe and efficient development while averting possible consequences, such as diastasis recti or episiotomy recovery. Here's how to tweak your regimen to get the best outcomes:

Rectus diastasis:
Put stability first: Give special attention to workouts that work your deep core muscles (transverse abdominis, pelvic floor, and so on) without using your rectus abdominis. Simple pelvic tilts, birddogs, and supine leg lifts with bent knees are a few examples.

Don't do sit-ups and crunches: These workouts may exacerbate the separation since they immediately engage the rectus abdominis.

Be mindful of your posture: Throughout the day, keep your posture correct to maximize core activation and aid in recovery.

Seek expert advice: See a physiotherapist with expertise in diastasis recti for guidance on appropriate exercise and progression.

Ectopic Recuperation:
Begin slowly: After speaking with your doctor, start out with low-impact activities like swimming, strolling, or mild yoga positions.

Put your attention on strengthening your pelvic floor. Kegel exercises are a must for regaining muscle tone and promoting recovery. Contractions should begin briefly and deliberately, then be progressively lengthened and intensified as permitted.

Pay attention to what your body tells you and steer clear of any activities that make it hurt. If you feel like it's ripping or tugging, stop.

Include scar tissue massage: Scar tissue may be made softer and less sensitive with a gentle massage using oil or specialty lotions.

Seek expert advice: A pelvic floor physical therapist may evaluate your condition and suggest exercises based on your individual recovery goals.

Overall Advice:
Warm up and cool down: To avoid injury, always warm up before an activity session and cool down afterward.
Preserve appropriate shape by prioritizing quality over quantity. It's crucial to use good form while doing workouts to prevent further straining or pain.
Rest and recuperate: In order to heal and avoid setbacks, enough rest and recuperation are essential.

Like any other attempt, Kegel exercises need persistence and progress monitoring to be successful. The following advice can help you keep on course and recognize your accomplishments:

Monitoring Development:
Maintain a record: Keep a record of the date, the quantity of Kegel sets and repetitions, the length of the contractions, and any emotional notes you may have in a notebook or app.

Make use of visual assistance To see your development over time, make a graph or progress chart. This is particularly beneficial for maintaining motivation.

Take measurements or pictures: Keep note of the number of spills or mishaps that occur before and after beginning Kegels exercises if you have specific objectives in mind, such as better bladder control.

Employ biofeedback To get visual or audio feedback on the contractions of your pelvic floor muscles, think about getting biofeedback equipment. This might assist you in making sure you're doing the exercises properly and getting the most out of them.

Maintaining Motivation:

Establish attainable objectives at first, then progressively raise them as your strength increases. Rejoicing in little victories can help you stay inspired.

Locate a partner for accountability: Tell a friend, relative, or medical expert about your objectives so they can encourage you and keep you on track.

Make it enjoyable: Find enjoyable methods to include Kegel exercises into your everyday routine. While doing them, experiment with various postures, use weights or Kegel cones to push yourself, and listen to music.

Treat yourself: Treat yourself to something non-food to celebrate your accomplishments, such as a massage, a new exercise attire, or a leisurely evening out.

Pay attention to the advantages: Remind yourself of the benefits of your work, such as less discomfort, or better control over your bladder.

Setting realistic objectives and maintaining a Kegel notebook might be effective strategies for achieving success in your pelvic floor strengthening journey. How to maximize them is as follows:

Kegel Journal:
Monitor your advancement: Keep a record of the date, the quantity of sets and repetitions, the length of the contractions, and any feelings you had both during and after the Kegel exercise session.

Keep an eye on changes: Observe trends and advancements throughout time. Did you leak less frequently? Do contractions have more force? Honor even little victories!

Determine obstacles: Keep a record of any challenges you have, such as missed sessions, soreness, or trouble activating your muscles. This might assist you in troubleshooting and routine modification.

Remain responsible: Keeping a journal of your accomplishments might serve as a source of inspiration and support for you.

Make use of prompts: You might include reflective parts like "What goals do I want to achieve this week?" or "How motivated am I feeling today?"

Creating Reasonable Objectives:
Start modest: Start with small, manageable objectives, such as doing three sets of ten Kegel exercises each day.
Concentrate on consistency: Kegel exercises are best performed often for little periods of time rather than seldom for prolonged periods of time.
Give specifics: A quantifiable, time-bound aim may be, "Increase contraction duration to 8 seconds by next month."
Honor significant anniversaries: Reward yourself for your progress to maintain your motivation.
Adapt as necessary: Don't be scared to adapt your objectives in response to your

advancement or any modifications to your situation.

Writing Advice for Journals:

- Make use of a notepad or a Kegel app.
- Select a format that is comfortable for you, such as tables, charts, or free writing.
- Don't overcomplicate things or get bogged down in details.
- Regularly go over your diary to keep on course and recognize your accomplishments.

Chapter 3
Enhancing sexual function with kegel Exercise

Arousal, desire, lubrication, orgasm, and overall pleasure are just a few of the characteristics of sexual function that are influenced by a complex interaction of physical, emotional, and psychological variables. In addition to supporting pelvic organs and aiding in sexual function, the pelvic floor muscles are essential for controlling bowel and urine movements as well as sexual activity.

Robust and synchronized pelvic floor muscles improve a number of sexual functions, such as improved sensation, increased blood flow, and regulated contractions of the muscles during an orgasm. Sexual function may be adversely affected by dysfunction, which can include muscular weakness, stiffness, or incoordination. Common problems include painful sex, trouble getting an orgasm, and diminished feeling as a result of uncontrollably weak or uncontrolled muscles.

By strengthening and toning the pelvic floor muscles, enhancing control over muscle contractions during orgasm, and improving blood flow and sensation in the genitalia, pelvic floor exercises—often referred to as Kegel exercises—can greatly improve sexual function. Good pelvic muscular tone, which is necessary for sexual function, is a result of strong pelvic floor muscles. Robust muscles may improve arousal and libido, improve blood flow to the vaginal region, promote arousal and responsiveness, and intensify and regulate orgasms.

Frequent Kegel exercises have a good effect on sexual function by maintaining or enhancing the health of the pelvic floor muscles. Seeking advice from a pelvic floor physical therapist or medical practitioner might be helpful if you have particular questions or concerns.

Higher blood flow, an improved orgasmic response, greater muscular control, support, and stability, improved vaginal tone, and higher confidence are just a few ways that stronger pelvic floor muscles may improve sexual sensation and enjoyment for both partners. Strengthening these muscles naturally and effectively may have a good influence on sexual sensation and pleasure. One such exercise is the Kegel.

Postpartum sexual problems are frequent, and managing them takes patience, open conversation, and even expert advice. Following childbirth, there are several strategies to address decreased libido and pain during intimacy. These include being open and honest with your partner, being patient and understanding, seeing your healthcare provider for postpartum checkups, engaging in pelvic floor exercises, taking care of lubrication, attending intimacy education, and concentrating on activities that foster emotional connection.

Recall that each person's experience is unique, so it's important to address postpartum sexual problems patiently and understandingly. If necessary, getting expert assistance may provide customized solutions for a more fulfilling and joyful personal life after giving birth.

Exercises like Kegels that strengthen the pelvic floor muscles may enhance vaginal tone, arousal, lubrication, blood flow, and the orgasmic response. A more appropriate supply of oxygen and nutrients are delivered to the vaginal organs by improved blood circulation, which is facilitated by improved muscular tone. This improves genital sensitivity and pleasure, which in turn increases total sexual enjoyment.

Engorgement of the erectile tissues and greater sensitivity in the genital area are supported by the increased blood flow to the genital area, which is a critical component of arousal. Additionally, it helps with better lubrication, which lessens dryness and pain during sexual activity, particularly for newborn females.

Robust pelvic floor muscles have the potential to enhance climax intensity by facilitating improved regulation of orgasmic contractions. Exercises like Kegels help to enhance muscle tone and coordination, which makes it possible for orgasms to occur with more powerful contractions. Coordinated and powerful feeling is enhanced by controlled rhythmic contractions. More sensitivity makes the vaginal region more sensitive, which produces more focused and powerful orgasmic reactions.

By delaying the orgasmic release, people may prolong the exhilarating feelings that precede the climax. Enhanced pelvic floor muscle endurance is essential during intercourse because it allows contractions to last longer, resulting in a longer and more powerful orgasmic experience.

In conclusion, the regulation and force of orgasmic contractions are directly influenced by the strength of the pelvic floor muscles. Exercises that target these muscles, such as Kegels, have been shown to have a good effect on the general level of enjoyment and quality of sex.

Exercises for the pelvic floor called kegels have the ability to activate the neural pathways linked to orgasm. Increased blood flow, nerve sensitivity, pelvic nerve activation, nerve signal synchronization, and strengthening the neuromuscular link in the pelvic area are some of the ways that these simulations may take place.

Although the benefits of Kegel exercises may differ from person to person, many people report that they improve their sexual function. A fulfilling romantic relationship requires a regular and comprehensive approach to sexual health that incorporates exercise, communication, and general well-being.

Kegel exercises may provide a sense of physical control, which can help with orgasm control and increase overall happiness. Better timing and rhythmic contractions, greater pelvic floor muscle tone, improved muscular control during arousal, delayed release, a sensation of mastery, increased endurance, and a positive psychological effect may all help accomplish this. Regularly doing these exercises enhances one's physical health as well as their ability to handle their personal relationships with confidence and empowerment.

Kegel exercises that emphasize pelvic floor sensations may help increase awareness of genital feelings during intercourse. To strengthen the mind-body connection, intentionally contract and release the pelvic floor muscles. Because of the increased mind-body connection that results from practicing mindfulness, people become more sensitive to pelvic sensations.

Frequent Kegel exercisers may help develop heightened pelvic sensitivity, which may foster a greater awareness of and appreciation for the feelings felt during intimate times. People who are more sensitive may be more aware of the subtleties of touch and arousal during intimate situations.

A more sensitive and pleasurable sexual encounter may result from improved reaction to stimulus. A more responsive and pleasurable sexual experience may result from increased awareness of pelvic feelings, which may be achieved with Kegel exercises.

People who practice mindful presence during intimacy are more likely to be alert and in the moment during sexual activity, which facilitates a deeper connection with the feelings and sensations felt during intimate times. A more happy and successful sexual relationship may result from improved communication with a partner due to an increased awareness of genital sensations. This communication allows people to communicate their preferences and wishes.

To sum up, by concentrating on pelvic floor sensations during Kegel exercises, one may enhance their awareness of genital feelings during sexual activity, which can lead to a more profound and conscious experience of intimate moments.

Chapter 4

Optimizing Your Pelvic Health for a Lifetime of Wellness

Retaining a robust and healthy pelvic floor is essential for several areas of health, such as controlling one's bladder and bowel, promoting sexual function, and avoiding prolapse. The pelvic floor is supported and strengthened in large part by lifestyle choices.

1. Physical Activity: To maintain a healthy weight and improve general health, participate in frequent, moderate exercise. Exercises that strengthen and stretch the pelvic floor include yoga, swimming, and walking.

2. Low-impact workouts: Kegel exercises and other targeted pelvic floor exercises are crucial for building muscle directly. Aim for three sets of ten to fifteen contractions, many times a day.

3. Weight Management: To prevent undue pressure on the pelvic floor, refrain from high-impact exercises like heavy lifting and leaping. Instead, maintain a healthy weight.

4. Healthy Diet: Eat a diet high in fruits, vegetables, and whole grains as well as other fiber-rich foods to encourage regular bowel movements and avoid constipation, which may put pressure on the pelvic floor.

5. Fluid Intake and Bladder Habits: To stay hydrated, drink plenty of water throughout the day, stay away from things that irritate your bladder, and make sure you completely empty your bladder while using the restroom.

6. Additional Supportive Practices: Give up smoking, control your stress, keep your posture straight, and get aid from a professional if necessary.

Keeping your pelvic floor in good condition requires consistency. Including these lifestyle modifications into your routine, in conjunction with expert advice when necessary, may greatly enhance your pelvic floor health and general well-being. For individualized advice, it's best to speak with a healthcare provider if you have any particular pelvic floor issues or symptoms.

Pelvic health is highly impacted by a number of variables, including stress, food, exercise, and weight management. Consuming fiber encourages regular bowel movements and helps avoid constipation; on the other hand, being properly hydrated preserves tissue flexibility and helps with both bladder and bowel functions. Exercise helps to strengthen and increase the flexibility of the pelvic floor muscles. One such exercise is the Kegel exercise. Frequent exercise helps control weight and is good for general health. Reducing extra strain on the pelvic floor muscles, which may result in diseases like pelvic organ prolapse and urine incontinence, is possible by maintaining a healthy weight. Hormonal balance is regulated by hormone balancing, which is crucial for pelvic and reproductive health.

Muscle tension brought on by stress might result in pelvic pain and discomfort. It might be helpful to manage stress by practicing mindfulness and relaxation practices. Hormonal changes during menopause and the prostate may have an influence on health, but pregnancy and delivery can also have an impact on pelvic health. Prostate health may be supported by regular exercise and a diet high in fruits, vegetables, and antioxidants.

Pelvic health may be impacted by inflammation and allergens, so controlling diet and recognizing possible triggers can be helpful. Positive impacts on pelvic health may result from a comprehensive strategy that takes stress, nutrition, exercise, and weight control into account. Optimal pelvic health is a result of leading a healthy lifestyle that includes a balanced diet, frequent exercise, managing weight, and reducing stress. Seeking advice from medical specialists is crucial for receiving individualized treatment and managing certain issues or symptoms.

Your pelvic health is greatly impacted by four important lifestyle factors:

1. Fiber-rich foods: To thicken stool and ward against constipation, consume 25–35 grams of fiber per day. Incorporate whole grains, legumes, fruits, and veggies into your diet.

2. Hydration: To avoid constipation and maintain the health of your bladder, drink plenty of water throughout the day. Reduce your intake of acidic beverages, alcohol, and caffeine to lessen bladder irritation.

3. Exercise: Consistently engaging in moderate-intensity physical activities like yoga, swimming, or walking strengthens the muscles of the pelvic floor and enhances general health.

4. Weight control: To lessen undue strain on the pelvic floor, maintain a healthy weight. Avoid unhealthful weight reduction methods and strive for a healthy body mass index (BMI).

5. Stress management: Techniques like deep breathing, yoga, and meditation may help lower stress levels and enhance pelvic floor tone.

Other recommendations for promoting long-term pelvic floor strength and function include stopping smoking, keeping proper posture, and forming healthy behaviors. Regular pelvic floor exercises (kegels), keeping a healthy weight, drinking enough water, eating a balanced meal, doing cardiovascular activity on a regular basis, and adopting a mindful posture are all important practices to support pelvic health.

Choosing gentle exercises that are friendly to the pelvic floor, managing chronic cough, seeking professional guidance for pelvic floor physical therapy, practicing stress management techniques, monitoring pelvic health during routine health checkups are all examples of ways to improve pelvic floor awareness and pelvic health. You can maintain the strength and function of your pelvic floor over the long run by incorporating these healthful routines into your daily routine. Seek the advice and assistance of healthcare specialists, such as pelvic floor physical therapists, if you have any particular concerns or symptoms pertaining to pelvic health.

Massage, yoga, and mindfulness are examples of complementary treatments that may greatly enhance pelvic floor health. By assisting people in releasing tension from their pelvic floor muscles, mindfulness techniques help people feel less stressed and more at peace. Tension may also be released with the use of yoga, which focuses on strengthening and extending the pelvic floor muscles. Yoga breathing exercises, like pranayama, may improve breath awareness, which helps ease tension in the pelvic floor and encourage relaxation.

When massage therapy is administered by licensed professionals, it may help the body relax and recover by releasing tension in the muscles and increasing blood flow. The goal of pelvic floor physical therapy is to enhance pelvic floor function by relieving muscular tension via a comprehensive approach that includes stretches, exercises, and manual treatment. It is individualized care that targets certain problems to provide the best outcomes.

Pelvic floor muscle relaxation may be aided by breathing techniques including diaphragmatic breathing and synchronized breathing with movement. Through the use of real-time feedback on muscle activation, biofeedback treatment enables patients to see and manage their tense muscles. Heat treatment may also aid in muscular relaxation and pain relief; it is often used in combination with other relaxation methods.

To make sure these procedures are customized to each patient's requirements and situations, it is crucial to check with healthcare specialists since individual reactions to these treatments may differ. Complementary treatments may enhance relaxation, function, and general well-being when included into a holistic approach to pelvic floor health.

A vital aspect of delivery is postpartum parenting, and new parents may find a range of tools and support systems to assist them in adjusting to this new role. A few of these resources are exercise classes, sleep support, pelvic floor rehabilitation, online platforms and apps, parenting classes, breastfeeding support, family and friends, books on postpartum wellness, postpartum doula services, online communities, professional counseling services, and self-care techniques.

Postpartum support groups provide a forum for establishing connections with other new parents, exchanging personal stories, and obtaining emotional assistance. During the postpartum phase, doula services may provide knowledge on infant care, practical aid, and emotional support. Parenting and postpartum health books may provide insightful advice. Online forums are a great place to talk about postpartum experiences with other women.

For those who are having trouble adapting or who are suffering from postpartum mood disorders, professional counseling services may be helpful. Postpartum care, infant care, and adapting to parenthood are some of the topics covered in parenting seminars or workshops. Lactation consultants and breastfeeding support groups are good resources for information about breastfeeding. In addition to providing emotional support and communication, family and friends may also serve as a supporting network. Exercise courses may help you progressively resume physical activity, and tools like safe co-sleeping or creating a regular sleep schedule can help you learn more about sleep support.

For people who are having problems with their pelvic floor after giving birth, pelvic floor therapy may be helpful. Apps and web platforms may provide community forums, information, and tailored advice. Self-care techniques, such setting aside time for oneself, are critical to general wellbeing.

During the postpartum phase, it is essential for wellbeing to have an optimistic attitude and recognize accomplishments. To overcome obstacles and keep a positive outlook, try acknowledging small victories, being grateful, setting reasonable goals, exercising self-compassion, organizing milestone celebrations, interacting with others, accepting imperfection, giving self-care activities top priority, celebrating personal development, keeping track of accomplishments, and consulting a professional.

In conclusion, managing the postpartum phase is an important aspect of giving birth, and it's critical to locate tools and assistance that meet your requirements. You can guarantee a happy and successful postpartum experience by embracing imperfections, prioritizing self-care, celebrating personal growth, documenting accomplishments, connecting with others, practicing self-compassion, setting reasonable expectations, appreciating small victories, and getting professional advice.